THE CHOKING PERIL

ndersen Young Readers' Library

Hazel Townson

THE CHOKING PERIL

Illustrated by David McKee

Andersen Press · London

First published in 1985 by
Andersen Press Limited,
20 Vauxhall Bridge Road, London SW1V 2SA

© Text 1985 by Hazel Townson
© Illustrations 1985 by Andersen Press Limited

Reprinted 1986

This edition first published in 1999

British Library Cataloguing in Publication Data available

ISBN 0 86264 930 7

Printed and bound in Great Britain
by the Guernsey Press Company Ltd.,
Guernsey, Channel Islands

Contents

1 Seeds of an Idea   7

2 A Budding Crime   16

3 Blooming Fireworks   24

4 A Bunch of Trouble   31

5 A Flowery Speech   46

6 A Thorny Problem   51

7 Turning Over a New Leaf   60

8 Wreaths and Smiles   69

For the Codd super-family of Newark
Pauline, Mike, Debbie, Stewart, Emma and Nicky

1
Seeds of an Idea

'There's far too much litter about,' grumbled Arthur Venger. 'Just look at my garden, filled with bus tickets and lolly sticks and toffee papers. As for the pavement outside my gate, it looks like the end of a market day.' He began stuffing into a huge plastic bag the disgusting objects which lay strewn around. One screwed-up newspaper, smelling of chips; one rotting carrot; two squashed Coke tins; three cigarette packets; four apple cores . . . .

Just as he reached out for a particularly nasty-looking hunk of mouldy bread, young Kip Slater said, 'I thought you were working on a cure for litter-dropping?'

Kip and his friend, Herbie Coswell, had come to call on Arthur in the hope of being able to help with one of his experiments. For Arthur Venger was a unique combination of chemist, inventor, salesman and crusader, bent on trying to improve the world. With this improvement in mind, he usually had some sort of experiment on the go. The boys had become involved with one of these experiments at their last school Speech Day, and were now Arthur's devoted admirers.

'I *have* worked on lots of cures for litter-dropping,

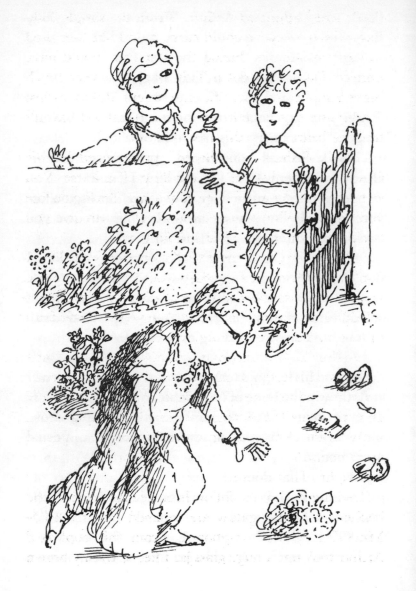

that's true,' admitted Arthur. 'From the simple Tidy Bag, which everyone could carry round like they used to carry gas-masks during the last war (you'll have noticed *I've* always got a Tidy Bag) to a very much more complicated scientific experiment. But as my last Truthpaste experiment was such a disaster, I haven't had the heart to try this new one out.'

'Well, I think you should,' pronounced Herbie Coswell the genius. 'It's like falling off a horse. You should get back on again straight away, before you lose your nerve. What you need is somebody to give you back your confidence. We can do that.'

'I'll say we can!' agreed Kip enthusiastically. 'I don't honestly think Tidy Bags would catch on. People wouldn't be bothered. But a real scientific experiment is a different matter. Let's try it! We've got terrific faith in you, and six weeks' holiday to spare.'

Arthur looked unconvinced, but at that moment a car drew up alongside his bit of pavement, the driver opened the door, tipped out the contents of his ashtray on to the space that Arthur had just cleared, then drove away again. Arthur flung down his bag in disgusted amazement.

'Right! That does it!'

Inviting the boys to follow him, he marched into the kitchen of his bungalow and opened the EXPERI-MENTAL ONLY cupboard. From this cupboard Arthur took out a huge glass jar filled with tiny brown seeds. 'These,' he explained importantly, 'are the seeds of my very own, incredible, fast-growing weed which I've christened Litterwort. That Litterwort will spring up fast and furious wherever it happens to fall. It creeps. Well, no; it doesn't so much creep as *gallop*! It will roam over concrete and marble and plastic and glass. In fact, there's only one place it won't grow, and that is where I've sprayed my other equally staggering product, ALIWOS.' Here, Arthur produced an object like an orange-coloured hairspray can and waved it in the air.

'Anti-Litterwort-Spray, of course,' Herbie the genius translated before Kip had even begun to wonder what ALIWOS meant.

'Now,' continued Arthur, 'what we have to do is *punish* the litter-droppers. If they can't see that litter makes a mess of their town, perhaps they'll see that Litterwort *does*. If we could manage to put these seeds into likely bits of litter, then spray the insides of *litter bins only* with ALIWOS, I think we would soon be able to teach the public better manners. With thick weeds growing everywhere and choking everything up, they'd have to stop and think. Especially since we'd also put up posters everywhere, saying: LITTER BREEDS LITTERWORT. YOU STOP THROW-ING—THE WEEDS STOP GROWING.'

'NO WEEDS GROW IN—A LITTER BIN,' added Kip, who had not been christened Kipling for nothing.

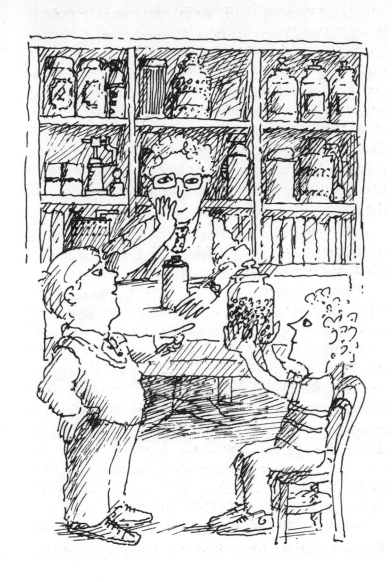

'H'm! Not a bad idea!' pronounced Herbie thoughtfully. 'There'd always be enough busybodies to take up the challenge and bully everyone else into being tidy. Your main problem, of course, would be getting your seeds into the public's hands. You'd better leave that to us. We'll distribute them for you.'

Kip looked sceptical. 'Do you mean to say we'd have to put one of these seeds inside every cigarette packet, every toffee paper, every lump of orange peel...?'

Herbie sighed. 'Use your brains. How could we? What we would have to do is fix our own special items of litter. Give out something which people are likely to throw away. We could have a flag day, for instance. Every flag folded double with a seed inside it.'

'That wouldn't work,' retorted Kip. 'Most of the people I know who buy flags—(and that's not many these days)—hang on to them like Superglue so they won't have to buy another. My Uncle Colin even saves his Remembrance Day poppy and irons the petals for next year.'

'Then he's tighter than a thumb-screw and doesn't deserve to live in a free country,' Herbie sneered. 'But I suppose you're right—flags are not really litter.' He pondered further until inspiration struck again. 'All right then, free gifts! With seeds in the wrappers. When folks open the gifts and throw down the wrappers they throw down the seeds as well.'

'Free gifts? That's going to cost us a fortune.'

'It needn't. I've got a drawer at home stuffed full of free gifts from cornflake packets, soap powder offers, etc. So have you, Kip. Then there's the stuff we got for presents and didn't want. Toys we've grown out of.'

'People are going to be mighty suspicious if we just start giving things away,' warned Arthur. 'They'll think there's a catch in it and refuse to take one. I knew a man who stood on a street corner once for a bet, offering real fivers for sale at 50p each, and nobody would buy one. They didn't want to look foolish.'

'But suppose we had a good reason for giving things away?'

Herbie's face suddenly glowed. 'Grumpton Carnival!' he cried, referring to an annual event that was due in a few weeks' time. 'You could dress up as Father Christmas, Mr Venger, and give out presents then. People would think it was all part of the Carnival fun. Kip and I could be your helpers. Reindeer or something.'

'I'm not being the back half of a reindeer.'

'All right, snowmen then.'

'H'm!' mused Arthur. 'It might just work. The Carnival procession starts and finishes in the park, and Bert Higgs, the Park Superintendent, told me he'd had to move fifteen tons of litter after last year's Carnival. If we gave out the presents there, it would be a good start to our plan. The Litterwort would soon take hold in the park. And we could stick our posters on all the gates, seats, fences and shelters.' He rubbed his hands with growing excitement. 'I'll buy some real gifts, too. May as well do the thing properly. I'll get my money back in the end, because people will have to pay me to spray my ALIWOS, and I intend that to be mighty expensive.'

Arthur began a list of all the things they would need. 'One—presents. You bring what you can—(good quality stuff, mind; nothing damaged or dirty)—then leave the rest to me. Two—wrapping paper; sheets and sheets of it.'

'I'll take care of that,' Kip volunteered. 'My mum saves all the paper off our Christmas and birthday presents ready to use again. She has a suitcase full.'

'What a family!' sneered Herbie. 'Does she iron that as well?'

'Waste not, want not!' Kip retorted loyally.

'Three—a Father Christmas outfit,' continued Arthur. 'That can be hired. Maybe the snowmen's costumes can, too. If not, we could easily make something out of papier-mâché and cotton wool. As for the posters, we'll work on those together.'

'We're in business!' cried Herbie. The triumphant gleam in his eye was a beacon to banish holiday boredom.

'Pity about the park, though. I rather like it,' mused Kip. 'I can't fancy the swings and boating pool and rose garden all thick with horrible weeds. Not to mention the bandstand and the bit where we play cricket.'

'Well, don't forget we can soon put things to rights when people have learned their lesson,' Arthur Venger reassured him. 'A huge dose of ALIWOS and all will be well. See what it says on the ALIWOS spray? "It kills as it spills." Litterwort only, of course.'

'It slays as it sprays,' improved Herbie.

'It slaughters as it waters,' capped Kip. 'Bags I the ALIWOS spray to squirt round the litter bins.' But Arthur said he had better do that bit himself, as mistakes at this stage would be fatal.

A slow grin spread itself across Arthur Venger's face, and his bright blue eyes began to twinkle. 'I'm going to enjoy every minute of this!' Little did he know how wrong he was.

2

A Budding Crime

'The best day for a robbery,' said Mungo Slye, 'is Carnival Day.' He tapped with the tip of his pencil at the spot on his map where Grumpton Museum was marked. Mungo had already ringed this spot in red.

Perce O'Deary looked worried. 'But Mungo,' he complained, 'the museum's right opposite the park. That's where the Carnival procession starts and finishes, and after that there's the fair and the band and the fireworks and I-don't-know-what, all in the park. Everybody will be there.'

'Exactly!' Mungo smirked. 'Plenty of riot, noise and hullabaloo! Just what we need to cover up our little bit of business. Furthermore, all the police will be otherwise engaged, keeping the Carnival crowds in order.'

'But the Carnival's on Bank Holiday Monday. The museum will be closed.'

Mungo cast his eyes towards the ceiling and said in long-suffering tones, 'I suppose you expected us to walk into a museum full of people and make our snatch with everybody watching?' Really, Mungo sometimes wondered why he didn't take hold of Perce O'Deary and shake him until his dandruff went into orbit. Mungo had to remind himself that he needed an

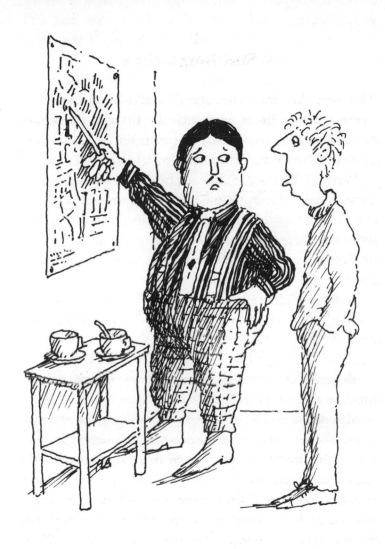

assistant who was not bright enough to realise what was going on, especially the value of the loot involved. Mungo must try to be nice to Perce until the whole daring plot was safely carried out.

'Carnivals mean dressing up. Fancy costumes,' explained Mungo patiently. 'That suits us fine. We'll dress up as burglars, with check caps and black eye-masks and sacks stuffed with newspaper, saying SWAG in big, red letters. Then we'll mingle all afternoon, so that everybody sees us. When they see us again at night with the real swag, they'll take no notice.'

'Mingle?' Perce echoed doubtfully. He didn't know what mingle meant, but guessed it had something to do with the Carnival Morris dancing. Mungo had asked Perce if he was light-fingered. Should he have said light-footed?

'We'll mix with the crowd,' said Mungo slowly, as if to a child of three. 'We'll walk about the park and enjoy ourselves, like everybody else. Then when it's dark and the fireworks start, we'll slip round to the back of the museum. I'll deal with the burglar alarm while you keep watch, just like we practised yesterday. Then I'll cut out a window-pane and Bob's your uncle. I'll be in and out again in fifteen minutes with the Baron in my sack.'

Perce peered through a fog of bewilderment. At last he muttered: 'But Mungo, my uncle's called George.'

Mungo ground his teeth, yet forced himself to grin,

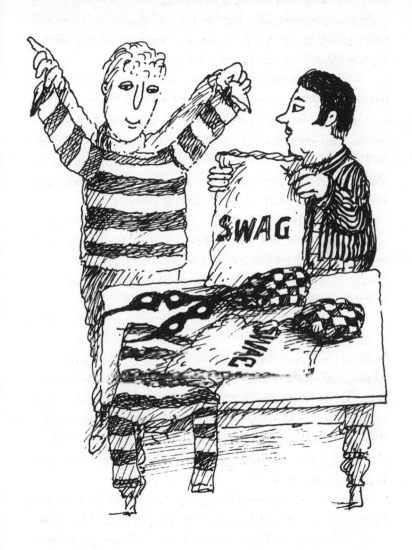

giving Perce's shoulder a soothing pat.

Of course, Mungo did not intend to stuff a real, live Baron into his sack; only the Baron's wax bust which had been set up in the museum by a grateful Town Council. For Baron Banks was Grumpton's most illustrious inhabitant. Not only had he become world famous for his invention of the micro-celery-silencer, thereby turning himself almost overnight into a millionaire, but he had then bestowed his riches liberally on the town, providing a swimming pool, a museum and two new football pitches, as well as fountains, flagpoles and floral displays galore. The bust, proudly placed in the entrance-hall of the new museum, was the expression of the townsfolk's gratitude.

Some people might think that a wax bust was a strange thing to steal. Yet there was method in Mungo's madness. Mungo worked as a clerk in a solicitor's office, and had been given the job of filing away Baron Banks's will. Being a naturally inquisitive person, Mungo soon discovered two sensational facts. Firstly, that Baron Banks had secretly bought the magnificent Eyeball Diamond, one of the rarest jewels in the world, so-called because it resembled a human eyeball in shape and size. Secondly, that the Baron, who was fond of practical jokes and had no family of his own, had bequeathed this diamond to 'the Grumptonian who manages to find it first', thus promising to set in motion a splendid treasure hunt after his death. Naturally, so far nobody knew about all this except the Baron, his solicitor and Mungo. The solicitor was as good at keeping secrets as a doctor or a priest. He would already have shut out of his mind all details of the Baron's will, which gave Mungo a head start in the treasure hunt. The will did not say *when* the diamond should be found. So why wait until Baron Banks's death, by which time there would be thousands searching for it? The moment to find it was *now*.

Being a well-trained villain, Mungo kept his eyes and ears open at all times, ever ready to profit from the folly, greed and carelessness of other people. For instance, he had spent a great deal of time in Grumpton museum, trying to decide which objects were worth stealing. Whilst there, he had gradually come to notice that when the sun was in a certain position, so that its rays fell through the stained-glass window on to the Baron's bust, the eye behind the monocle winked and sparkled in a strange and lively way. Far too strange or lively for glass or plastic. Could this be the vital clue?

It was well known that the eccentric Baron often visited his bust, whispering in its ear and patting it on the head. He could so easily, on some quiet Monday morning, have gouged out the plastic eyeball from behind the plastic monocle and substituted the Eyeball Diamond, suitably painted over with a dark brown eye.

At any rate, that was Mungo's guess. Now he could

prove himself right. What a coup it would be to steal the Eyeball Diamond! What a feat of intelligence and daring! And what a smart way to ensure that Mungo could live happily ever after without doing another stroke of work! No more nine-to-five sessions in a dusty office. No more putting up with thick-headed messenger-boys like Perce O'Deary, who always got everything wrong and left Mungo to take the blame. Nothing but peace, leisure and luxury for ever!

Mungo knew that if he was to break into the museum, he needed a look-out . . . somebody who would not guess what he was really up to. The perfect candidate was Perce O'Deary, the world's most muddled non-thinker, who could easily be persuaded that Mungo was 'borrowing' the bust as part of a charity rag, to raise money for the local Children's Home. The museum would have to buy back the bust by giving money to the Home, he told Perce.

'Nothing in it for us, of course. We're just helping the kiddies.'

Perce, who had been brought up at the Children's Home, thought this was a great idea.

Mungo's first plan had been to prise out the precious diamond from its socket. On second thoughts, he decided he might scratch and damage it. Anyway, prising it out might take too long. Better to steal the whole bust instead. Baron Banks's bust would just fit nicely into the sack marked SWAG. And since the

Baron was at present away on a world cruise, no one would realise the significance of the theft until Mungo had got clean away.

3
Blooming Fireworks

The day of Grumpton Carnival dawned bright and windy—just the right weather for scattering seeds. Crowds converged upon the town from miles around. Full car parks, traffic jams and pavements packed with procession-watchers turned the town into a simmering pot of trouble. Pick-pockets, handbag-snatchers and vendors of reject balloons wove in and out upon their villainous errands. Toni's Ices doubled their prices. Harpo's Hot Dogs shrank to half their usual size. Yet none of this seemed to dampen the festive spirit. People were determined to enjoy themselves and to forget their everyday cares. For weeks, all had looked forward to this event, and they jolly well intended to make the most of it, especially the free presents from Father Christmas and his snowmen. Something for nothing! That was the way to set the fingers grabbing!

'Pink for girls, blue for boys, purple for grown-ups. Only one each *please*, madam! I don't care if you *have* got forty-nine grandchildren. And please put your litter in the bins, or you'll start a plague of weeds.'

It took less than an hour for Arthur and his helpers to dispose of a bulging sackful of presents, and dozens of screwed-up wrappers were already bowling merrily

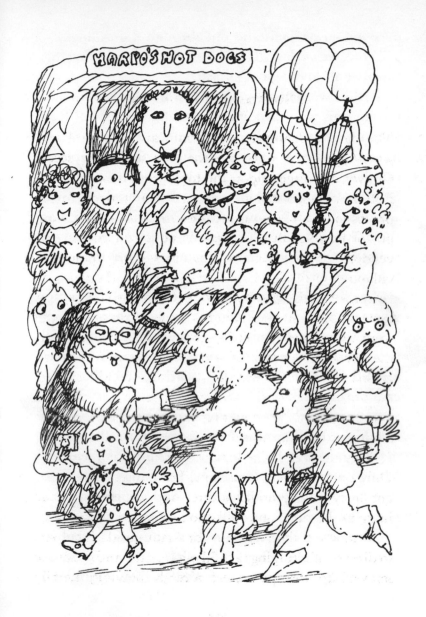

over the flower-beds and out through the railings.

'Well, we've done it now! By tomorrow morning this town won't know what's hit it!'

Arthur went back to his car for a second sack-load, pushing his way through a colourful mixture of Red Indians, pirates, fairies and Romans. He even met a human giraffe, a walking toadstool and a couple of burglars. Arthur had to chuckle at the sacks marked SWAG. One good thing about the annual Carnival was that it brought out people's ingenuity as well as their litter. 'In fact, this year,' chuckled Arthur to himself, 'they'll get more ingenuity than they ever bargained for.'

The fireworks began at nine o'clock in the evening, when the sky was dark enough to show them at their best. Grumpton Carnival was famed for its wonderful firework display, and heads turned upwards from miles around to watch the winking, soaring, crackling patterns of colour.

Mungo Slye's head was no exception. He, too, was watching the fireworks from a spot near the park's main gates, but he was not watching for pleasure. Mungo was waiting for the bigger bangs to start, so that he could set about his thieving. A noise to hide a noise, as Mungo's mother used to say when young Mungo turned up the radio volume to cover the crunch of his shop-lifted toffees.

Stars burst and rockets fizzed and flew. Pink and

26

blue balls cascaded on to tree-tops and away on the skyline Mungo could see the Carnival bonfire glowing orange and red at the other end of the park.

At last there came a great explosion, followed by an upward thrust of sparks. Then crack-crack-crack, and bang, and boom, and crack-crack-crack again. Now was the moment! Mungo grabbed Perce's arm and hurried him away through the upward-gazing crowd, out of the park gates, across the road and round to the back of the museum. The cobbled back street was deserted. The museum sat dark and silent in the middle of a row of closed-up banks and shops and offices. Setting down his sack, Mungo shook out all the screwed-up newspapers he had filled it with, then folded the sack, stuffed it inside his jacket, and began work very gently on the burglar alarm.

Perce, his head still reeling with the fireworks, took up his post at the end of the back street, supposedly keeping watch. But every time another rocket shot into the air, so did Perce's gaze. A blind old woman could have picked Perce's pocket and he wouldn't have noticed.

At last, Mungo had the window out. He set the pane down gently on the pavement, then climbed in through the gap, groping his way carefully until he felt it was safe to switch on his torch.

It seemed a long way round to the entrance hall at the front of the building. For a while, Mungo thought

27

he must have taken a wrong turning, but he came out at last in the high-windowed hall where the bust of Baron Banks had pride of place. A sudden firework flash lit up the room, and Mungo saw clearly the Baron's waxen head with its thick, white hair, its moustache, its monocle—and behind the monocle its fiercely sparkling eye. It was an eerie sight. There was Mungo, alone in that silent room, with an eye that seemed to be watching every move he made. A good thing Mungo was not a fanciful man! He found it much more natural to think of all the things he would be able to buy with that Eyeball once he had sold it. Top quality hand-sewn suits; regular subscriptions to all the comic papers; a set of fishing tackle; a bungalow with gnomes and a goldfish pond; a blue-and-green-striped sports car . . . .

Now he had actually reached the pedestal on which the bust stood. Now he had his hands round the Baron's slippery, waxen throat. Whoops! He almost dropped it! But at last he had the Baron safely in his sack, and was making his getaway.

When Mungo reached the empty back window-frame, he checked that Perce O'Deary was still standing at the end of the road, exactly where Mungo had left him. Yes! Good lad! He was still there . . .but wait a minute! What was Perce O'Deary doing? He was actually standing there chatting to a policeman! The policeman had interrupted his beat to spend a com-

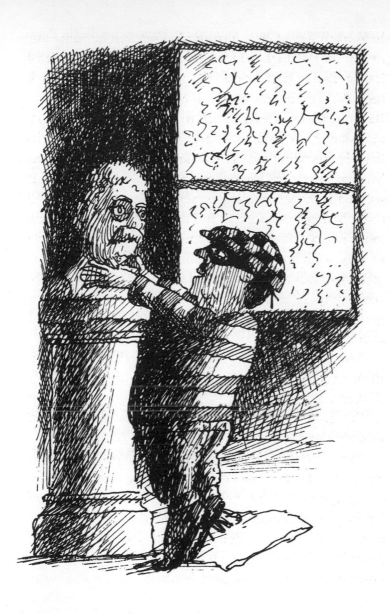

panionable moment swapping comments with Perce about the novelty of Perce's costume and the quality of this year's fireworks. The two of them were getting on like a colony of ants.

Mungo stepped back in alarm. For a while he hid and waited, his poor heart banging as hard as a coffin-maker's hammer in a plague.

The policeman showed no signs of moving on. In fact, he had taken quite a fancy to Perce, who was wondering whether to tell him about the charity rag. Mungo decided he would have to let himself out by the front door and run off in the other direction. He had seen a bunch of keys hanging up in the Curator's office. Snatching these up, he tried every single one in the front door lock, without success. That meant he would have to remove another pane of glass and climb out by one of the front windows. 'Let's hope nobody's watching!' thought Mungo. 'Not that I've any choice.' Mungo had just removed this second pane of glass, thrown his laden sack through on to the pavement outside, and put one leg over the sill ready to follow the sack, when Perce's friendly policeman appeared in the hall.

'Now then, what's all this?'

Mungo was caught, and it wasn't even a fair cop. It was all Perce O'Deary's fault. One day Mungo would throttle Perce—but not for a while yet, by the looks of things.

4
A Bunch of Trouble

Arthur Venger set his alarm clock for the very crack of
dawn. By then the Litterwort should have grown quite
well, and Arthur wanted to be the first to see the results.
Kip Slater and Herbie Coswell had also arranged to
wake up early, so that Arthur could pick them up in his
car on the way to the park. After all, the lads had
helped with the presents, and with the pasting-up of
posters after dark, so they deserved to be in on the fun.

Arthur yawned and stretched, touching his toes
three times rather creakily before parting the curtains.
At first all seemed right with the world, but when he
rubbed his eyes and looked again, he saw that even
here, such a long distance from the park, weeds were
already springing up in the cracks between the pavings
and starting their forward crawl. One particularly
savage clump had climbed half-way up a wall and had
already obscured the LITTER BREEDS LITTER-
WORT sign. A better result than Arthur had hoped
for! Chuckling delightedly, he dressed, gulped down
his cornflakes and coffee, then hurried to his car. This
would teach everyone a lesson, and no mistake.

Arthur lived on the outskirts of Grumpton, but as he
drove nearer to the centre of the town he found the

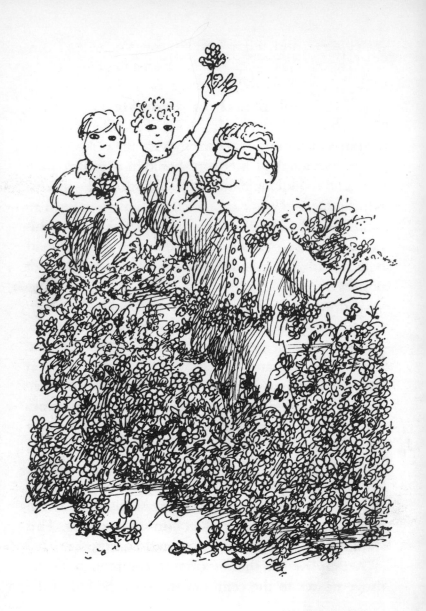

going more and more difficult, for patches of ever-thicker and more tangled weeds loomed in his path. In some places it was like trying to drive through a blackberry bush. By the time he reached the road where Kip and Herbie lived, he was having a very bumpy ride and decided to leave his car and walk. Of course, Arthur had brought with him a can of ALI-WOS and could have cleared a patch for himself if he had wanted to. But that would have made things easier for everyone else as well, and you don't teach people a lesson by making things easier for them, Arthur reasoned. So Arthur stepped out of his car.

At once, a strange thing happened. Arthur took a deep breath—and stood entranced! What was that wonderful smell? He breathed again. The smell seemed even more wonderful. Not a smell, but a perfume, a rich, sweet, magical scent that made him feel totally happy. For quite a few moments he could do nothing but stand and draw in deep lungfuls of the heady stuff, smiling with closed eyes at the wonder of it all.

A perfumed weed! The Litterwort was perfumed! This was something Arthur had never even thought of. In the experimental stages, he had grown only one or two shoots of the stuff, and as he had had a cold at the time he had never noticed any perfume. But this! Why, it was a miracle! If it made everyone feel as happy as he felt at this moment, then it must be worth a fortune. It was even prettily coloured; most pleasant to look upon.

33

Six petals on each opening flower were ranged in alternate pinks and yellows and blues. Greedily, Arthur plucked a bunch of Litterwort and held it to his nose. He strewed it on his car seat, stuck it in his buttonhole, his belt, his pockets. He was almost delirious with joy.

This was how Kip and Herbie found him, having spotted Arthur from the top of Kip's garden wall, which they had had to climb because the gateway was choked with weeds. The boys were already over-excited.

'Some weed, Mr Venger!'

'Why didn't you tell us it would be like this?'

'I didn't know!' breathed Arthur, shaking his head incredulously. His brain buzzed wildly with the new possibilities. Here was not merely something to clog up the roads and create a nuisance. Here was a positive contribution to the quality of life, as valuable as fine food and drink, good holidays, great music, paintings, poetry. Not what Arthur had intended at all.

Herbie had seen a few possibilities, too. 'This stuff must be worth a fortune! A pity you didn't just grow yourself a gardenful, Mr Venger, so you could have sold it. Now it belongs to everybody. It's theirs for the picking.'

'We could go round with the ALIWOS spray,' suggested Kip, 'and kill it all off. Then start again, just planting seeds in Mr Venger's garden.'

34

Arthur shook his head, dispelling the daydreams.

'That wouldn't do much to solve the litter problem, would it? And anyway, it would take far too long. The world would be astir long before we'd finished.' Indeed, it was already too late, for as he spoke a nearby door opened and a sleepy Fred Jepps, the local milkman, began to amble slowly up a weed-strewn path on his way to the dairy.

Fred was more than usually tired this morning, having stayed late at the Carnival the night before. In fact, he felt quite stupefied with weariness, and stopped in mid-pathway to rub his eyes and yawn. Then all of a sudden Fred Jepps woke up. He sniffed. He turned his head and sniffed again. He took a deep breath, like a diver about to plunge from the top board. At last he swung round and headed back to the house, calling excitedly to his wife: 'Hey, Millie, something's happened to our garden!'

'There you are!' commented Arthur sadly. 'Ten more minutes and the whole town will know.'

'Ten minutes!' groaned Herbie. 'That's all it takes to lose a fortune!'

Mungo Slye had also lost a fortune. He had been whisked off to the police station hours ago, without a chance to recover the bust in the sack. As far as he knew, it still lay there, on the pavement, waiting for the first passer-by to pick it up. Perce O'Deary's policeman

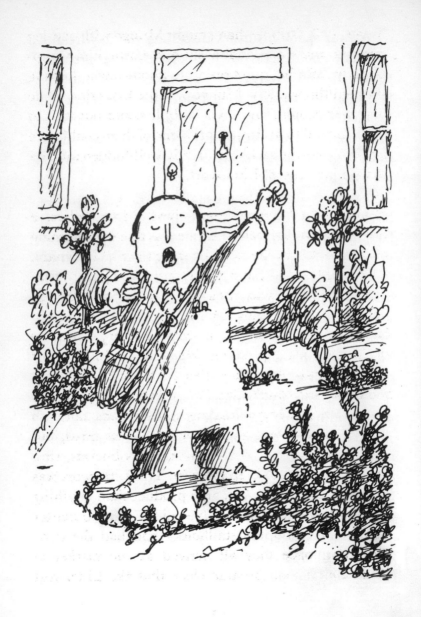

friend, P.C. Dribble, had caught Mungo with one leg over the museum window-sill and borne him triumphantly off for questioning without even looking through the window. Mungo was the first criminal he had ever caught, and P.C. Dribble could not wait to show him off to his Inspector. None of them could have guessed that the sack was already well-hidden under a thickening crop of Litterwort.

Next door to the milkman lived Eddie Sellars, a travelling market trader. Eddie was due that morning at the market in the neighbouring town of Lyckham. Eddie sold second-hand books; dog-eared paperbacks, musty old tomes with their backs hanging off, and so on. But today, hearing the racket made by his neighbour and quickly taking in what had happened, he decided to switch products. He would sell Litterwort instead. Eddie kept this idea to himself, but great minds began to think alike. Other Grumpton stallholders awoke, and began loading up their vans, not with rolls of cloth or antiques or vegetables as usual, but with great bunches of Litterwort, plus buckets, tins, vases and basins to keep them in. This Litterwort was suddenly a far more valuable product than anything they had ever sold before. Nor did it seem to matter that every Grumpton stallholder had had the same idea. For, once they all arrived at the market in Lyckham, it soon became clear that the Litterwort would go faster than free fritters in a famine. The cost rose from 50p a bunch to 50p a sprig. Then £1 a sprig, then £2, £5, £10—what a ridiculous way to make a fortune!

The news—and of course the wonderful smell—spread far and wide, and Lyckham market place was soon jammed with people. Some drove in from as far as a hundred miles away, having been telephoned by friends. Some moved like zombies in a trance, sniffing with closed eyes and great smiles of bliss. Fantastic sums of money were offered for the fragrant weeds, and the minute any stallholder sold out all he had to do was to rush back to Grumpton and pick another batch.

Arthur Venger, who had seen what was happening and followed the crowd to Lyckham, was now seized by a new worry. The whole thing was getting out of hand. He had not foreseen that people would actually *want* the Litterwort and carry it off to places where he would never be able to reach it.

'We must stop them buying it!' he cried distractedly to the boys.

So Herbie and Kip, misunderstanding, went around whispering in people's ears, telling them that they had no need to buy the stuff; they could just drive another couple of miles up the road and they would be able to pick it for themselves.

There was instant pandemonium. Cars drove off by the dozen, honking and swerving in the race to be there

38

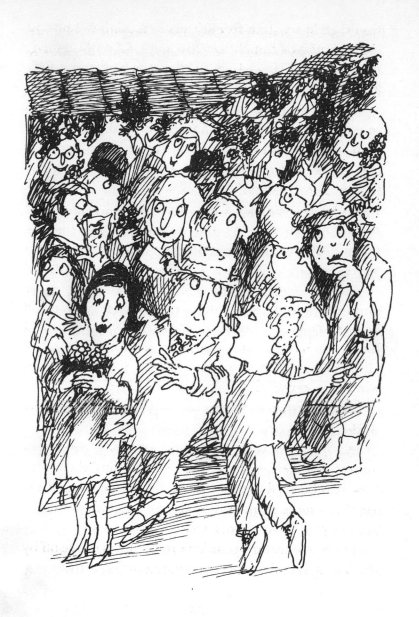

first. Soon the road into Grumpton became hopelessly jammed. Vehicles were abandoned where they stood, and drivers ran the rest of the way, leaping ecstatically at last into knee-deep verges of Litterwort. There, seized with a greedy madness, everyone began plucking and wrenching and sawing with penknives at the tough young stems. The mass of busy, bending bodies eventually pushed its way right into the centre of the town.

Now came the chaos which Arthur had intended, yet it came not from surging weeds, but from surging weeders. Every street was blocked with people. Innocent townsfolk could not even open their own front doors to nip and grab a bit of Litterwort for themselves. It was outrageous! Something would have to be done!

The telephone wires hummed with frantic messages, and at last, with enormous difficulty, the Mayor and a few of the councillors managed to make their way to the Town Hall for an emergency meeting. They all agreed that they couldn't put up with this state of affairs, but what was the solution?

'We'll have to push back these crowds and close off the town!'

'Nonsense! This is wonderful for trade!' retorted a councillor who happened to own a couple of supermarkets. 'All these pickers are getting hot and tired and thirsty. They'll need drinks and snacks and ice-creams and lunches and carrier-bags and bundles of string and sticking-plasters and picture postcards and I-don't-know-what. We've never done such good business for years.'

'It's no use making a fortune if you don't live to enjoy it,' observed the Mayor. 'Half the Grumptonians are going to be trampled to death at this rate. And what if a fight breaks out? It only needs A to lurch into B, and B to push him off, and you've got a riot on your hands.'

'Well, the answer is simple enough. If we get rid of these weeds the crowds will go. Can't we put some lawnmowers on to the roads? Or bulldozers or something?'

'Here, not so fast! Have you lost your sense of smell, or what? This stuff is the best thing that has ever happened to us. If we use our brains now we can make a fortune . . . .'

'Those who have *got* any brains can surely see . . . .'

At this moment the door of the Mayor's parlour burst open and a hot, dishevelled Arthur Venger appeared, waving a bag of seeds in one hand and an ALIWOS spray in the other. Arthur was a man with a conscience. When he felt he had done wrong he was anxious to confess and take his punishment. Kip and Herbie knew this, but felt that such impulsiveness would only lead to further trouble. They both came panting in behind Arthur, trying their best to restrain him.

'It's all my fault! I'm the one to blame!' Arthur shouted guiltily, and before the boys could stop him he had poured out the whole tragic tale.

'It's not really his fault,' objected Herbie. 'You can't stop weeds from growing if they want to.'

'It's everybody else's fault, for not putting their litter in the bins,' agreed Kip. 'You've seen what it says on the posters.'

'What posters?' asked a man who never read such things, on principle.

'Thought they were just a Carnival joke,' said someone else. 'Or the work of cranks and nutters. Plenty of those about these days.'

The Mayor, desperately trying to make sense of all this, began to remember a certain Speech Day at St. Bede's school, which he had attended some weeks ago. There had been some very funny goings-on at that Speech Day, and surely this was the man who had claimed responsibility? In which case, nothing was impossible, especially if these were also the same two lads who had been mixed up in the trouble. The Mayor pushed forward a plant-pot containing a wilting geranium. Plucking the geranium from the soil, he offered the pot to Arthur. 'Fast-growing seeds, you say? Go on then, give us a bit of proof. Let's see for ourselves.'

Arthur dropped a handful of seeds into the pot and pressed them down with his fingers. The Mayor watered them with a little can which he kept on top of his

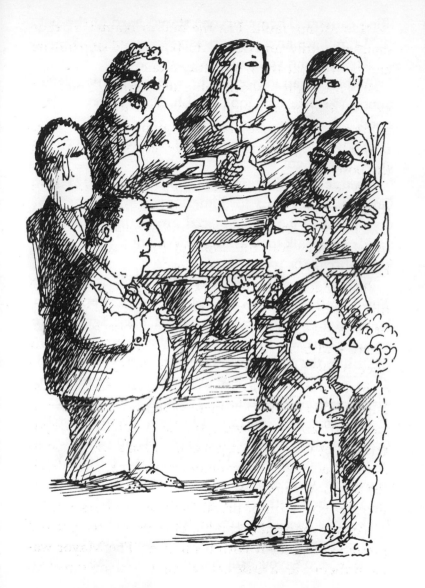

filing cabinet. Then everyone stared hard at the pot.

'I don't see anything growing.'

'He's having you on!'

Arthur began to sweat. These people seemed determined to make him look foolish. If only they understood!

'We can't stand about all day, waiting for seeds to grow. We've got a crisis on our hands.'

Distractedly, Arthur mopped his brow, and Herbie Coswell, feeling sorry for him, stepped into the breach, crying: 'Give it time! No seed grows that fast. Even Jack's beanstalk took all night. Why don't you have a coffee-break, or something?'

So that was what the party did, mooching off to the Town Hall canteen with sceptical faces. Yet half an hour later, when they all trooped back again, sure enough there was the tip of a tiny shoot showing above the soil in the pot. The Mayor bent over it. He sniffed. Then a great smile spread across his face, multiplying his chins from two to four.

'Let that be a lesson to all of you! Always give the benefit of the doubt. Without my restraining influence you'd all have gone rushing off, and we'd never have known we were sitting on a gold mine.' He turned to the wretched Arthur and slapped him heartily on the back. 'My boy, I'm proud to know you! You're a greater asset to this town than Baron Banks himself.'

'But don't you understand...?' began Arthur

desperately, only to be shouted down by the Mayor's firm reasoning: 'What's to stop you spraying a ring of that ALIWOS stuff round Grumpton? Then we'd be sure the Litterwort would grow nowhere else but here. We could cultivate it properly and charge outsiders to come and smell it. In nice, orderly queues, of course.'

'We could use the ALIWOS to clear the roads, and just let the stuff go on growing in the park,' cried someone else.

'I think you're forgetting something,' said Herbie Coswell the genius at the top of his voice. 'That Litterwort has already been sold at Lyckham market, to all sorts of people living outside the town. It's been carried off in cars for miles and miles. The seeds will scatter everywhere. The whole country—nay, probably the whole world—will soon be covered in the stuff. We are quite possibly witnessing the end of civilisation as we know it!'

'Cor!' said Kip.

5
A Flowery Speech

Inspector Lobb took another bite of his salami sand-wich.

'Now look here, Mungo,' he said with his mouth full, 'I'll be honest with you. The town's so crammed with crowds of crackpots today that things are a bit disrupted. We've not been able to get back into the museum to find out where you hid that bust, or even whether anything else is missing. So if you could see your way to *telling* us all about this little escapade, and saving us a lot of fuss and bother, then I could quite likely see my way to ordering you another salami sandwich. Maybe even an apple pie as well.'

Mungo's mouth began to water. He was absolutely ravenous. One salami sandwich went nowhere at all in a frame the size of Mungo's, and apple pie was his especial favourite. Besides, the SWAG sack was sure to have been picked up by now. It was probably on its way to being handed in at this very police station at this very moment. So where was the harm in confessing? He needn't say anything about the Eyeball Diamond, of course, and once he got out of here the bust would have been returned to the museum and there would be nothing to stop Mungo having another go at snatch-

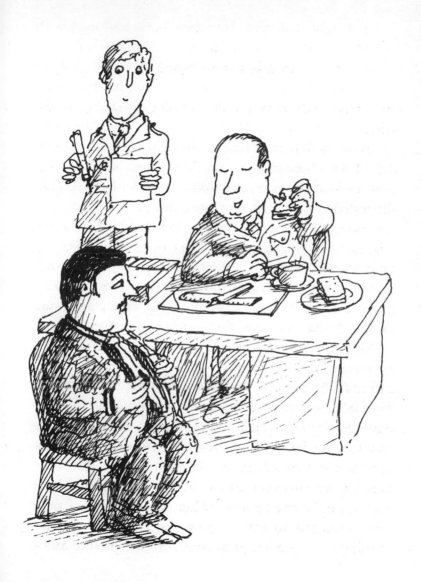

ing it.

'All right, you win, Inspector!' cried Mungo with seeming reluctance. 'I'll make a full confession.'

At a signal from the Inspector, Constable Dribble perched his notebook on his knee and licked his pencil as Mungo began: 'Hero worship, that was the start of it all. A rare disease these days, but a bad one. Once you suffer from that, you're a lost soul.'

Inspector Lobb's lip began to curl. 'Come off it, Mungo! The day anyone takes you for a hero, I'll eat shredded sweaty socks for breakfast.'

Mungo's eyes grew round with innocent wonder.

'Oh, not me, Inspector. I'm just the humble worshipper. Baron Banks is the hero. You see, I've always admired what he did for this town, and wished I could do half as much myself. Only there's one little snag about giving away a fortune—you have to *have* a fortune to start with. Me, I'm broke. So I thought of this charity stunt, to make money for the Children's Home. I'm sure the Baron wouldn't have minded his bust being borrowed for such a good cause.'

'Well, you do surprise me, Mungo! Are you asking me to believe that you're nothing but a sentimental old idiot after all?'

'Exactly, Inspector!' agreed Mungo, managing to wet his finger and drag it across his cheek like the path of a fallen tear.

Later that night, Constable Dribble was sent along

to look for the sack. With Mungo's instructions it did not take him long to find it, despite the weeds. Then he had the pleasure of dragging the Curator back to the museum from a comfortable after-dinner nap, to identify the bust.

The Curator was not pleased. He had spent a draughty day with two missing window-panes, and as a result he now had rheumaticky twinges in his shoulder. Also, the bust was damaged. One of its eyeballs was missing.

'The person responsible for this vandalism will have to pay,' he told Constable Dribble. 'The thing looks ridiculous with only one eye.'

The Constable was bound to agree that it did. Still, the Curator ought to be thankful for small mercies. The whole head could have been kicked to pieces by the mob.

The Constable failed to notice that there was a hole in the bottom of the SWAG sack . . . a hole more than big enough to let an eyeball through.

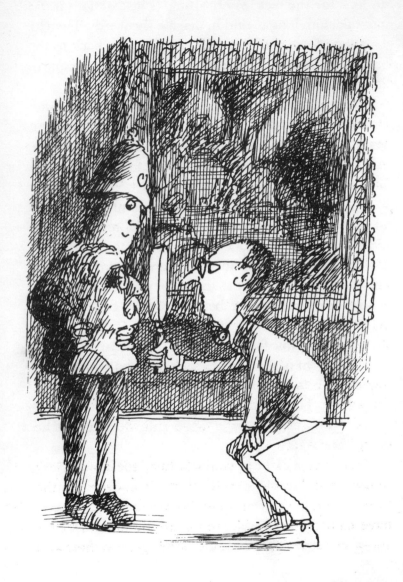

6
A Thorny Problem

After a totally chaotic meeting, the Mayor and councillors finally reached agreement. Arthur Venger must
spray all the weeds with ALIWOS as fast as possible
and kill them off, in spite of the perfume, which the
Mayor now referred to tearfully as 'a luxury we must
learn to do without'. Herbie Coswell's prophecy had
shaken him to the shoelaces. 'We'll get *our* town
cleared. The rest of the world will have to take care of
itself. Mind you, I'll send a warning telegram to the
Prime Minister.'

'Mention the ALIWOS,' the Town Clerk urged.
'There's still a chance we can make a fortune out of
that.'

'You mean Mr Venger can!' cried Herbie and Kip
together. Arthur himself was still too upset to do more
than wring his hands and moan.

'It's his invention, and if he doesn't want to use it he
doesn't have to.'

'Now, you look here, young laddie,' the Town Clerk
rounded on Herbie sternly, 'I don't know what the
three of you have been up to, but *you* are the ones who
have caused the trouble, so *you* are the ones who are
going to put it right. So you'd better get out there and

51

start spraying before you find yourselves in *real* trouble.'

'We did warn you! We put all those posters up,' cried Kip. 'You could have stopped this happening if you hadn't all been so lazy and careless and lackadaisical.'

'And we're not spraying anything,' retorted Herbie stoutly, 'until we're sure you're going to pay for it.' He had recently read *The Pied Piper of Hamelin* and felt he knew all about cunning, treacherous mayors and corporations.

'Kip, just pass me a sheet of that paper over there.'

Kip selected a page or two of the Mayor's best headed notepaper, upon which Herbie began to print a message in bold capitals: WE AGREE TO PAY ARTHUR VENGER WHATEVER HE SHALL REASONABLY DEMAND FOR SETTING TO RIGHTS THE WEED CRISIS IN GRUMPTON.

'Right! Sign that, all of you, one after another, or Mr Venger won't spray anything at all. Will you, Mr Venger?'

'Er—no,' squeaked Arthur. Then, taking courage from Herbie's evident command of the situation, he said more loudly and firmly, 'No, I jolly well won't!'

'That's the stuff, Mr Venger,' whispered Kip encouragingly. 'Never let yourself be browbeaten!'

'*And* you!' cried Herbie, spotting a councillor who was trying to slink from the room without signing. At last, when he was satisfied with the contract he had drawn up, he folded it carefully, stuffed it inside his shirt and ushered out Kip and Arthur.

'Where's that ALIWOS, then? Better get started right away.'

'It's going to take ages,' moaned Kip. 'Can't we get some help?'

But Herbie insisted they must do it all themselves. He wasn't going to let any Tom, Dick or Harry loose with Mr Venger's sprays, particularly with a fortune at stake.

'We'll manage. Just keep moving, that's the thing. We'll finish the park by teatime.' Arthur, inspired by Herbie's bossy confidence, had now perked up enough to take charge of the operation. He unlocked the boot of his car, which was full of ALIWOS cans, and the spraying began.

So hard did the three of them concentrate that they scarcely noticed the shouts and shufflings of the greedy crowds around them. Luckily, the crowds did not realise that the three were trying to kill off the Litter-wort, or there would probably have been a massacre. Most thought Arthur and the boys must be watering the weeds, or dealing with the greenfly, and they even cheered them on.

They sprayed until it was nearly dark and they were quite worn out. Even then, they had only just finished the park. All those roads and streets and gardens were

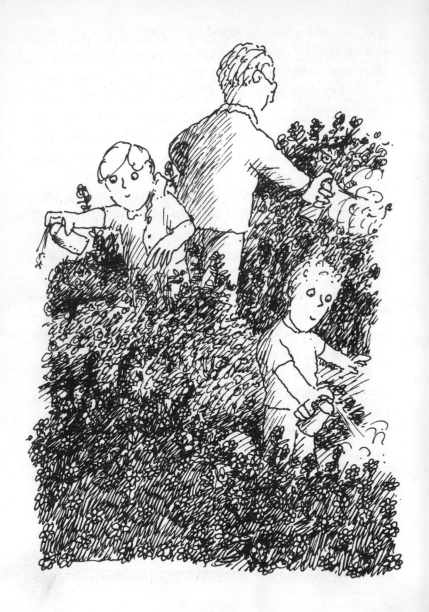

still to do. Yet their weariness was as nothing to their horrified dismay as they finally began to realise an awful fact. The ALIWOS did *not* kill the Litterwort after all! On the contrary, wherever they had sprayed, the weed looked and smelled more wonderful than ever, and continued to grow a good deal faster. The whole park was fast becoming a dense, unmanageable jungle.

They couldn't believe it! Everything had depended on the ALIWOS, and it had let them down. Arthur's guilt and remorse returned in double measure.

At last, they went home to Arthur's bungalow in despair.

'What am I going to do?' Arthur sank down dejectedly at the kitchen table, head in hands. 'Not only am I a failure and a laughing-stock, but I've probably ended the world.'

'You must have got it wrong,' pondered Herbie thoughtfully. 'When you made the ALIWOS you must have put in a wrong ingredient or something. Suppose we were to make another lot of ALIWOS and change the proportions?'

'You don't know what you're suggesting!' Arthur wailed. 'There must be about a million permutations. You could go on for ever, and spend a fortune, and still not get it right. It took me five years to come up with this.'

'Well, let's sleep on it. We'll all feel better in the

55

morning. Herbie and I must go home now, but we'll be back first thing tomorrow to help you again.'

'I wouldn't blame you if you never came near me any more.'

Steeped in self-pity, Arthur gloomily watched his guests depart. Then he slumped down across the table again and wished that he would die. Why was it that whenever he had a wonderful, earth-shattering idea, he had to go and spoil it with a bit of silly carelessness? 'It's a flaw in my character,' the little red-head told himself woefully. 'I really need a couple of assistants to keep a check on me. But nobody would want to work with a failure like me. I wish I'd never been born!'

Ten minutes later the boys were back. There was a great, excited commotion as they rushed in without knocking.

'Mr Venger, Mr Venger, the others are all dead!'

Arthur sat up with a jerk. What did they mean? Was he a mass murderer now? Had the entire population of Grumpton succumbed to the sweet but deadly perfume? No, no; that couldn't be right, or he and the boys would be dead themselves. Then what . . .?

'The other Litterwort—the lot we *didn't* spray with ALIWOS—the stuff in the streets! It's dying off by the ton!'

'It must only last a day or so!'

Arthur sat up even straighter. Then he stood up, whacking the table wildly. 'Wow! Do you realise what

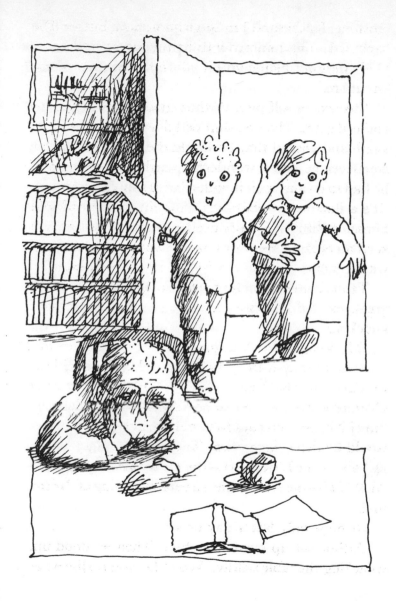

this means?'

'Of course!' replied Herbie promptly. 'It means this isn't the end of civilisation after all, but the start of a wealthy, famous Grumpton.'

'And a wealthy, famous Arthur Venger,' added Kip.

'All that stuff sold at the market will have died, as well. And as the ALIWOS spray seems to keep the Litterwort *alive,* we can have our parkful for as long as we want it.'

'We'll tidy it up a bit, of course.'

'Clear the paths, and so on.'

'Charge admission.'

'Enjoy the perfume ourselves—even up here at the bungalow if the wind's in the right direction.'

'It's a miracle!' Arthur cried at last. 'Do you realise that if I hadn't got it wrong . . .?'

'Just goes to show,' Kip broke in eagerly, 'that it's an ill wind that has no turning.'

'Of course, I can't expect the Council to pay me now, but never mind.'

'Oh, yes you can! I was very careful how I worded that contract. It didn't say anything about killing off; it only mentioned "setting to rights the weed crisis in Grumpton". Well, you've done that, so they'll have to pay up.'

'Herbie, you're a genius!' cried Kip unnecessarily.

'That was nearly a disaster, though. I think we'd

have been better off with the original Tidy Bags, after all. Tell you what, I'll give that idea a try for a day or two and see what I think of it.'

Herbie plunged his hand inside his shirt to draw forth the famous contract—and discovered that he'd lost it! Somewhere out there it was just another piece of litter.

7
Turning Over a New Leaf

Nobody has bad luck all the time. As if the Fates were determined to console Herbie Coswell for the loss of his contract, it was he who found the Eyeball Diamond as he pushed his broom through heaps of withered Litterwort. By this time, the Eyeball was covered in dirt and it was difficult to tell what it might be. Herbie guessed at a marble, and thought he might clean it up some time and give it to Kip, who collected them. But right now he was busy helping to clear the town. He slipped the Eyeball Diamond into his home-made Tidy Bag and forgot all about it.

Days passed; days in which Arthur and the boys had not time to think of anything but the Litterwort. With the help of Bert Higgs, the Park Superintendent, and his army of gardeners, Grumpton park soon became a tidy place once more. The paths were left unsprayed, then cleared of dead weeds, and everywhere else the Litterwort had been pruned into order. It thrived in shapely flower-beds bordered with tiny coloured stones. It made great archways over gates, and threw up columns and cones of colour among the trees. And over all, the wonderful scent wafted its fan of happiness. Meantime, the refuse carts had been out in the

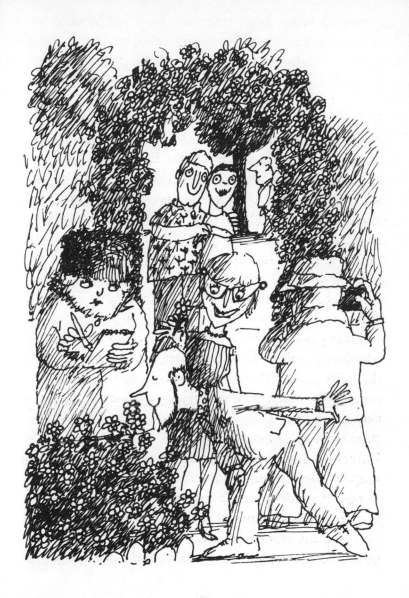

streets, clearing away the swept-up heaps of dead Litterwort. Paving stones were pushed back into place where spreading roots and shoots had forced them apart. The little town of Grumpton was coming back to life.

Back to a strange new life. For by now, of course, Grumpton's fame had spread across the whole country and beyond. Pictures of it were constantly seen on television news—(all channels). Visitors poured into the place to see—and more importantly, to smell—the Litterwort. Telephones never ceased ringing as long-distance callers tried to book rooms for a night, or a week or a whole summer. House prices soared. New tea rooms opened round every corner, and car parks in every spare bit of field. As far away as California, Grumpton-bound planes were being chartered, while in the depths of the Kremlin special agents were being briefed to sniff out this possibly world-threatening phenomenon. In short, Grumpton was on the map.

Grumptonians grew proud. Almost overnight, they developed a keen sense of loyalty to their hometown which was wonderful to behold. Instead of grumbling about the rotten bus service, the pigeon-droppings on the cenotaph and the lack of things to do on Saturday nights, they began to boast about the number of years they had lived in the place, and how many relatives they had in the local graveyard. They smartened themselves up in case some snooping television camera should catch them unawares; and for the same reason they washed their curtains, painted their front doors, tidied their gardens, mopped their steps and bought new dustbins. The place was practically unrecognisable. And all the time the wonderful perfume from the park filled everyone with joyful energy.

Yet, unlike the residents, the visitors had no pride in Grumpton. They didn't care about the town, except as a place to go for a picnic or a nice day out or a weekend away from work. Most of these visitors ate their lunches in the park, then threw down their empty bottles, tins, bags, packets, paper cups and plastic forks. Not to mention bus tickets, paper hankies, comics, camera-film cartons, toothpicks, disposable nappies, chewing-gum and a million other objects. Grumptonians grew more and more enraged. Here were they, slaving away to make the place look nice, and along came these uneducated louts who strewed their rubbish hither and thither without a moment's thought. It had to stop! (In fact, the Grumptonians began to feel exactly as Arthur Venger had felt when this story first started.)

The number of litter bins in the town was doubled, then trebled, with almost no effect. Great signs were set up, saying: DO NOT LEAVE YOUR LITTER HERE! but unseen vandals merely painted out the 'DO NOT'. At last, in despair, the Mayor called yet another emergency meeting, to which Arthur and his two young cronies were invited.

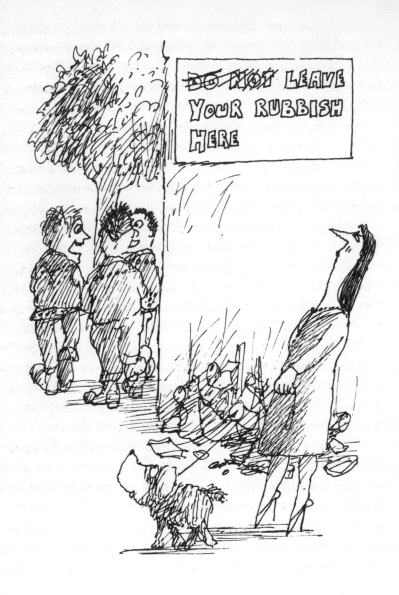

'Our town,' the Mayor pointed out, 'has become a remarkable place. It's unique. Everybody wants to see it. It's a showpiece, in fact. Well, the one thing about a showpiece is that it must always look its best. Same with princesses and such. You wouldn't want to see a princess with a ladder in her tights and black smudge on her nose and a hole in the elbow of her cardigan.'

'I wouldn't want to see *anybody* like that,' interrupted Herbie Coswell. 'Waitress or auntie or school-dinner-lady or whoever she was.'

'Yes, yes,' snapped the Mayor. 'Don't interrupt, please! You know perfectly well what I mean. It's the same with our town, I was going to say. From now on, our town must always look its best.'

'It was always the same with our town, even before the Litterwort,' boomed the great voice of Baron Banks, newly returned from his world cruise. 'I'll tell you this, I'm fed up with providing fountains and buildings and gardens that just choke up with litter. We shouldn't have had to wait for something like this to happen before we felt a twinge of pride.'

'Hear, hear!'

'Rubbish!'

'Nobody asked him to provide his fountains and gardens.'

'Well, that's gratitude for you!'

'He said he didn't *want* any gratitude. Last time he made a speech, he said . . . .'

The Town Clerk rapped on the table with his little hammer.

'Order, order! Those who interrupt this crucial discussion should have proper suggestions to offer.'

'Well, so we have,' cried Herbie, producing his Tidy Bag. 'If everyone carried one of these to put his litter in as he went about his business, then we'd have no problem at all. Mr Venger's been doing it for years.'

'It was the first of his ideas,' agreed Kip. 'If he hadn't realised that people were too jolly lazy to carry Tidy Bags, then he wouldn't have bothered inventing the Litterwort.'

There were shouts of scorn, disgust and disbelief, as Herbie drew back the strings of the little cloth bag he had been carrying for days. The shouts turned to howls of protest as, in order to demonstrate his point, Herbie began to take out the various items of litter, one by one, and lay them on the table. A screwed-up chocolate-wrapper; a burnt potato crisp; the crust off his lunch-time sandwich; a bit of gristle; a lump of bubble-gum; and—what was this? Something smooth and hard in the bottom of the bag, which Herbie now remembered he had not emptied for several days. The smooth, hard object was, of course, the Eyeball Diamond, now cleaned up from its constant rubbing against the side of the Tidy Bag.

At once, Baron Banks recognised the stone with its painted brown eye.

'The Eyeball Diamond! Where did you get that?'

'Diamond? A diamond as big as an eyeball?' Herbie's brain turned cartwheels, taking in this stunning news. Surely it was another miracle, which he must turn to the best advantage in order to prove his point.

'See what I mean?' he crowed. 'I picked that up as a piece of litter when it was dirty and unrecognisable. I had no idea it was a diamond. If my friend Kip here hadn't been a well-known collector of marbles, I'd have left the thing lying in the gutter. The rain would have washed it down a drain into the sewers, and we'd never have seen it again!'

Whereupon Baron Banks had a heart attack and fell down dead.

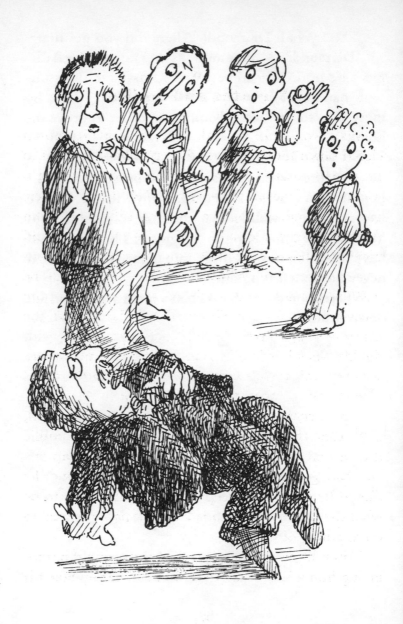

8
Wreaths and Smiles

It was a wonderful funeral. Everything in Grumpton closed down for the day, and every inhabitant, not to mention thousands of strangers, thronged the streets to watch the funeral procession. There were flowers galore, including a great cross of Litterwort from Arthur Venger, Kip and Herbie. There was a band playing solemn music all day, and black ribbons streamed from the top of every lamp-post. It would be true to say that the whole occasion was far more spectacular than the Carnival had been, and the *Grumpton Argus* gave it a full front-page spread, with double black border. The vicar, in his funeral oration, spoke of 'this town's great benefactor', and there was scarcely an eye that did not shed a tear.

But after the funeral came the reading of the will. And after the reading of the will came the public declaration that as Herbie Coswell, a true Grumptonian, had genuinely found the Eyeball Diamond, he should be allowed to keep it. That would seem to be what the Baron had intended. Herbie nobly refused to do anything of the kind.

'After all, it was me that killed the poor old Baron, giving him a shock like that. So I can hardly take his valuables.' No amount of reassurance by the Baron's doctor that the Baron had had a bad heart, and could have dropped dead at any moment, made the slightest difference. Herbie would not change his mind.

'What I *will* do,' said Herbie after careful thought, 'is to donate the proceeds from the sale of this diamond to a worthy cause. And the worthiest cause I can think of is the cause of progress towards a better world. Nobody I know has done more research towards that end than my friend, Mr Arthur Venger, who is always looking for cures for the ills of civilisation.' (Herbie saw this as his great chance to make up to Arthur for having lost that contract.) 'Of course, there will be donations, too, to our local charities, such as the Children's Home.'

There were great shouts and cheers among all who heard. (All except Mungo Slye, out on bail pending his trial for breaking and entering at Grumpton Museum.) Those who had felt jealous of Herbie's luck now gave him their ungrudging admiration, and Arthur Venger found himself a sudden hero. As for Perce O'Deary, no one had ever connected him with Mungo's crime, and as he didn't even know it was a crime he hadn't even a guilty conscience. In fact, he thought all this latest talk of money for the Children's Home was what Mungo had been arranging in the first place. Perce felt utterly happy, and quite proud of himself for having helped.

The reporter from the *Grumpton Argus* cornered

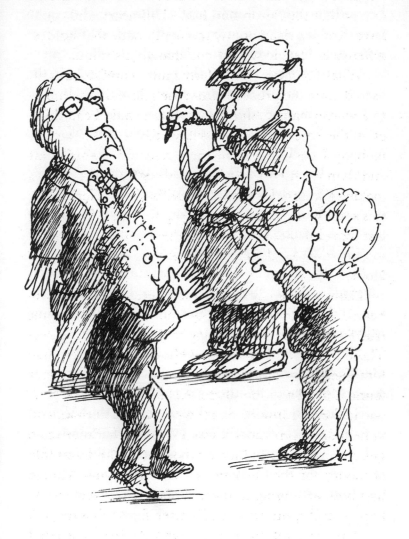

Arthur Venger to ask what sort of research could now be undertaken. Arthur's bright blue eyes began to twinkle. All his confidence had returned, and inspiration oozed from every pore. 'How about a Bore-Silencer?' he suggested, looking the reporter straight in the eye, 'to put an instant stop to all those people who ramble on and on about nothing . . . .'

'Including anyone who says, "I told you so!"' Kip amended gleefully.

'Or what about a Politeness Pill?' added Herbie.

'Or a Greed-Dissolver?' Kip went on.

'Or a Bad-Temper-Sweetener?'

'Or a Vanity-Watcher's mirror?'

'Or a . . . .'

'But of course,' declared Arthur as the list of suggestions grew, 'before I could undertake so much work I'd need an increase in staff. A couple of young assistants, say.'

Herbie looked at Kip, and Kip stared back at Herbie, who finally shook his head. 'It's no use. We're stuck with school for the next few centuries.'

Kip looked totally cast down, until Arthur Venger grinned and continued: 'Just evenings, weekends and holidays for a start, until the business really blossoms out in a few years' time. I'll tell you what, boys, if you're not doing anything tomorrow morning . . . .'

About the Author

Hazel Townson was born in Lancashire and brought up in the lovely Pendle Valley. An Arts graduate and Chartered Librarian, she began her writing career with *Punch* while still a student. Reviewing some children's books for *Punch* inspired her to write one herself. Over fifty of her books have so far been published and she has written scripts for television. *The Secrets of Celia* won a 'best children's book' prize in Italy and *Trouble Doubled* was shortlisted for a prize in the North of England. She also chairs the selection panel of the Lancashire Children's Book of the Year Award. Hazel is a regular visitor to schools, libraries and colleges and her books have been described as 'fast-moving and funny'. She is widowed with one son, one daughter and four grandchildren.

The Speckled Panic
Hazel Townson
Illustrated by David McKee

When Kip Slater buys *truth*paste instead of
*tooth*paste, he and his friend Herbie soon realise
the sensational possibilities of the purchase.
They plan to feed the truthpaste disguised in a
cake to the guest of honour at their school
Speech Day but, unfortunately, the headmaster
eats the cake first . . .

'A genuinely amusing quick-moving story'
British Book News

ISBN 0 86264 828 9
paperback

Hot Stuff
Hazel Townson
Illustrated by David McKee

After attempting to cure liars with Truthpaste
and litterbugs with Litterwort weed, inventor
Arthur Venger and his two young assistants, Kip
and Herbie, take on the hotheads – 'speed
maniacs, terrorists, football hooligans . . .' – in
an attempt to make the world a better and
more peaceful place to live. But as usual things
go disastrously wrong and the world ends up
anything but peaceful.

'Another pacy adventure from this entertaining
author'
Independent on Sunday

ISBN 0 86264 931 5
paperback

The One-Day Millionaires
Hazel Townson
Illustrated by David McKee

Arthur Venger, inventor of the notorious
'Truthpaste', has a brilliant new scheme to
make everyone feel more generous. But when
villains cash in on his idea to make a fortune
for themselves, chaos ensues.

'A funny and fast-paced story for fluent readers'
Independent on Sunday

ISBN 0 86264 835 1
paperback

Coughdrop Calamity
Hazel Townson
Illustrated by David McKee

Inventor Arthur Venger and his two young
helpers produce a cure for the common cold,
but they have reckoned without the
unscrupulous Bruno Kopman who will go to
any lengths to preserve his Comical Cough Sweet
business – (a joke on every wrapper). Also hot
on the trail is Doctor Yess who wants the cure to
sell to his rich Harley Street patients. Theft,
kidnapping, corny jokes and mayhem lead to a
devastating conclusion.

ISBN 0 86264 834 3
paperback

Disaster Bag
Hazel Townson
Illustrated by David McKee

Colin Laird is seriously worried about the state
of the world. Disasters are happening all
around him, and he decides to acquire a Disaster
Bag filled with all the equipment he might need
in an emergency. Only then does he begin to
feel safe. But how could he possibly guess that
a terrorist would slip a bomb into his bag when
he wasn't looking . . .?

'One of Townson's best'
Books for Keeps

ISBN 0 86264 524 7
paperback

Trouble on the Train
A Lenny and Jake Adventure
Hazel Townson
Illustrated by Philippe Dupasquier

On a train trip to a Manchester museum, Lenny
overhears a sinister-sounding conversation. Has
he stumbled across a plot to blow up the train?
He tries to pass on a warning, but nobody will
believe him. So he and Jake take matters into
their own hands, ending up in a life-
threatening situation from which they have to
be rescued by a *girl*!

This is the fifteenth story in Hazel Townson's
popular *Lenny and Jake* series. The last story,
The Clue of the Missing Cuff-link, was praised by
the *Independent on Sunday* as a 'fast, funny and
hugely entertaining read'.

ISBN 0 86264 624 3
paperback

TROUBLE DOUBLED
including
Dads at the Double and Double Snatch
Hazel Townson

Two exciting mysteries by Hazel Townson are combined in this paperback original.

Dads at the Double
After meeting at a Schools Drama Festival, Paul and Sara, who live at opposite ends of the country, begin a correspondence. But their letters gradually uncover a horrifying truth which could devastate the lives of both families.

Double Snatch
Angela's weekend visits to her estranged detective dad involve her not only in his case-load but also in a frightening drama which puts her best friend's life at risk.

'The action is artfully advanced through correspondence'
Daily Telegraph

ISBN 0 86264 710 X
paperback